HARVESTING HEALTH

Plant-Based Nutrition Secrets for Happy Families

Wholesome Vegetarian Family Meals for Optimal Well-Being and Vitality

Laura D. Vandergriff

ALSO BY LAURA D. VANDERGRIFF

- ➢ <u>**VITALICIOUS CUISINE:**</u> <u>**Heart-Healthy Recipes for**</u> <u>**Vibrant Living**</u>

- ➢ <u>**SIMPLE BUT POWERFUL**</u> <u>**GUIDELINES FOR**</u> <u>**KEEPING YOUR HEART**</u> <u>**HEALTHY**</u>

- ➢ <u>**REVERSE TYPE 2**</u> <u>**DIABETES IN 30 DAYS**</u>

- ➢ <u>**THE CALORIC RESET:**</u> <u>**Ignite Your Metabolism,**</u> <u>**Ignite Your Life**</u>

Contents

Introduction

Introduction

Get to know the Rodriguez family. With busy lives that didn't leave much time for home-cooked meals, the Rodriguezes fell into the trap of the modern diet, which is made up of fast food, comfort foods, and drive-thrus. They ended up with a lot of health problems because of it, ranging from mood swings and weight gain to long-term-illnesses.

But everything changed when they learned how powerful plant-based nutrition could be. The Rodriguezes started their plant-powered journey after hearing about other people who had changed their lives by changing their food and way of life. They cleaned out their kitchen, put bright fruits and veggies in the fridge, and promised to cook meals at home as a family.

The effects were nothing less than amazing. It only took a few weeks for their energy, happiness, and general sense of well-being to completely change for the better. The extra weight started to melt off, their skin lit up with health, and they felt full of life and happiness again.

But what the Rodriguezes may have found most important was something really deep: just eating together could feed not only their bodies but also their minds. They got to know each other better and made memories that will last a lifetime as they sat around the dinner table laughing, talking, and enjoying every-bite.

These kinds of stories tell us of the huge potential we all have—the potential to get our health back, change our lives, and make a future full of health, happiness, and plenty. And this idea is what keeps us going as we start this journey together.

Our health is something that often gets neglected in the busy world we live in now. Families have a lot going on between work, school, and other activities, so it can be hard to find the time and energy to make healthy eating a priority. But in the midst of the chaos lies a huge chance—a chance to change not only our own health but also the health of our whole family.

Imagine a normal morning at the Smith house. The alarm goes off, letting you know that another busy day has begun. Parents are in a hurry to set the table for breakfast, and kids are in a hurry to find backpacks and socks that match. In a busy world, ease often wins over health, and sugary sweets and processed snacks are the go-to foods to get you through the   day.

What if there was a better way? Think about what would happen if families could use plant-based nutrition to feed their bodies and souls instead of processed foods that are full of additives and-preservatives?

We go on just this kind of trip in "Harvesting Health." This book is full of useful information, ideas, and tips that will change the way your family eats and lives. We will talk about how plant-based eating can change your life, using both the newest nutrition studies and tried-and-true knowledge from countries all over the world. We will talk about everything from how it can improve your physical health to how it can bring your family closer together and help them be stronger.

1

"Grant food to be thy relentlessly solution be thy food."

The term "plant-based eating" has recently arisen as a prominent paradigm in the field of nutrition, and various experts have praised the benefits of this consumption pattern. Hippocrates, the man who is considered to be the founder of modern medicine, appropriately said that the meals that we eat have a significant influence on our health and well-being. In the modern world, when chronic conditions such as heart disease, diabetes, and obesity are quite common, adopting a plant-based diet provides a glimmer of hope—a way to achieve robust health and energy.

Evidence from the Scientific Community in Favor of Plant-Based Dietations

Research from the scientific community is largely in favor of the health advantages of eating a plant-based diet. Diets that are abundant in fruits, vegetables, whole grains, and legumes have been demonstrated to be related with decreased rates of chronic illness and greater lifespan, according to several studies. For instance, a meta-analysis that was published in the Journal of the American Heart Association found that adhering to a plant-based diet was related with a 25% decreased risk of developing heart disease [1]. In a similar vein, research that was published in the Journal of the American Medical Association demonstrated that plant-based diets are helpful for reducing body fat and improving metabolic health [2].

Considerations Regarding the Environment and Ethical Issues

Not only is a plant-based diet beneficial to one's own health, but it also has significant advantages for the planet and the people who live on it. The effect that animal husbandry has on the environment is startling, since it is a contributor to the destruction of forests, the polluting of water sources, and the release of greenhouse gases. On the other hand, diets that are based on plant foods have a substantially smaller carbon footprint and may contribute to the reduction of climate change [3]. In addition, adopting a plant-based diet is consistent with the ethical ideals of compassion and sustainability since it lessens the need for factory farming and significantly lessens the amount of pain that is caused to animals.

Practical Advice for Individuals and Families Looking to Make the Switch to a Plant-Based-Diet

It is possible that the process of switching to a plant-based diet as a family may first seem to be intimidating; nevertheless, with proper preparation and support, it can be a journey that is both gratifying and pleasurable. In order to assist you in making the move as seamless as possible, here are some practical tips:

1. *Commence with a gradual approach:* To begin, increase the number of plant-based meals that you include on your weekly menu. Explore new culinary creations and make a conscious effort to cut down on the amount of animal products you consume.

2. *Place an emphasis on whole foods:* place an emphasis on plant foods that are whole and have undergone little processing, such as fruits, vegetables, whole grains, nuts, seeds, and legumes. There is a broad range of health advantages that may be derived from these foods, which are abundant in vital nutrients.

3. *Encourage your creativity in the kitchen:* by experimenting with a variety of cooking techniques and taste

combinations to ensure that your meals remain both interesting and fulfilling. For the purpose of cultivating a feeling of ownership and enthusiasm about plant-based eating, it is beneficial to engage the whole family in the process of meal planning and preparation.

4. *Educate Yourself:* Make it a priority to educate yourself about the nutritional advantages of plant-based meals and the ways in which they may contribute to the overall health of your family. Put yourself in a position to make educated decisions about your nutrition by arming yourself with information and resources.

5. Remember that the move to a plant-based diet is a journey, not a destination, and that you should be *flexible in your approach.* You should be willing to try out new dishes and cuisines, and you shouldn't be too harsh on yourself if you make a mistake every

once   in   a   while.

In order to effectively embrace a plant-based diet as a family and successfully enjoy the many health and environmental advantages that it provides, it is necessary to take incremental steps and approach the shift with an open mind and a positive attitude.

A plant-based diet has a great deal of potential for the purpose of encouraging compassion for all living creatures, saving the earth, and increasing health. We have the ability to build a better and more sustainable future for ourselves and future generations by embracing the power of plants and making deliberate decisions about the foods we consume.

2

Understanding Nutritional Basics

When making the switch to a plant-based diet, it is particularly important to have a solid grasp of the foundations of nutrition since nutrition plays a significant influence in our general health and well-being.

Surprising Statistics Regarding the Deficiencies of Key Nutrients

As opposed to what is popularly assumed, nutrient shortages are more widespread than previously thought, especially in industrialized nations. Even while there is a plenty of food available, there is still a possibility that plenty of people, especially those who follow omnivorous diets, are lacking in key nutrients. On the other hand, persons who follow plant-based diets that are not well planned may have a higher opportunity of experiencing deficiencies. Surprisingly, research suggests that the following:

1. *Vitamin B12 insufficiency:* Research has shown that vegetarians and vegans have a high frequency of vitamin B12 insufficiency. The rates of vitamin B12 deficiency in vegetarian children range from 25 to 85 percent, while the rates in vegetarian teenagers range from 21 to 41 percent.

2. *Iron insufficiency:* is another major worry, especially among women and children. Iron deficiency is specifically an issue that affects women. Although the body is able to absorb iron from plant-based sources more easily than it can from animal-based ones, the danger of iron insufficiency is higher when using plant-based sources.

3. *Zinc and omega-3 fatty acids:* Vegetarians and vegans may also have difficulty reaching their zinc and omega-3 fatty acid needs, which are

predominantly found in foods produced from animals. Animal-derived foods are the primary source of these nutrients.

These data highlight the need of careful meal planning in order to guarantee an appropriate intake of critical nutrients, particularly when following a diet that is mostly composed of plant-based foods.

Foods derived from plants include a variety of essential nutrients. There is a multitude of critical elements that may be found in plant-based meals, which are crucial for good health and vitality. Plant-based diets, when carefully designed, have the potential to provide our bodies with all of the nutrients they need, contrary to the widespread belief. Here are some essential elements that can be found in abundance in diets derived from plants:

1. *Protein:* Legumes; such as beans, lentils, and chickpeas, in addition to

tofu, tempeh, nuts, and seeds, are all good sources of protein that come from plants. The consumption of a wide range of these meals guarantees that an appropriate amount of necessary amino acids will be consumed.

2. *Iron:* Although plant-based sources of iron are non-heme and less quickly absorbed than heme iron from animal products, integrating iron-rich foods into meals, such as lentils, spinach, tofu, and cereals that have been fortified with iron, may help satisfy daily needs for iron. The absorption of iron is improved when these meals are combined with alternatives that are high in vitamin C.

3. In addition to leafy greens like kale and collard greens, plant milks that have been fortified with *calcium*, tofu, almonds, and sesame seeds are some examples of plant foods that are high in calcium. For optimal bone health, make it a habit to consume these foods on a

daily   basis.

4. *Vitamin B12:* Because vitamin B12 is largely found in animal products, it is vital for persons who follow a plant-based diet to acquire this component via fortified foods such as plant milks, cereals, nutritional yeast, or by supplementation by consuming these items.

5. *Omega-3 Fatty Acids:* Flaxseeds, chia seeds, walnuts, and hemp seeds are all good sources of omega-3 fatty acids for those who adopt a plant-based diet. The consumption of these items on a regular basis helps to guarantee that a suitable amount of alpha-linolenic acid (ALA), which is a precursor to another omega-3 fatty acid, is consumed.

Instructions on Dietary Planning in Order to Achieve a Balanced Diet
In order to guarantee that every member of the family receives the necessary

nutrients while adhering to a plant-based diet, meal planning is essential. Here are some helpful hints for preparing meals that are both well-balanced and rich in nutrients:

1. *"Diversify Your Plate":* When you eat, try to include a wide range of colors, flavors, and textures into each meal. To ensure that you are getting a broad variety of nutrients, you should consume a variety of foods, including fruits, vegetables, legumes, nuts, and seeds.

2. *Give Whole Foods Priority:* When it is even somewhat feasible, choose whole foods that have undergone minimum processing. These are foods that are rich in nutrients and offer the body with the vitamins, minerals, and antioxidants that it needs.

3. *Incorporate Protein-Rich Foods:* Some examples of foods that are high in protein are beans, lentils, tofu, tempeh,

edamame, quinoa, and seitan. Maintaining muscular mass, promoting satiety, and assisting in a variety of biological activities are all benefits of consuming protein.

4. *Choose foods that have been fortified:* To ensure that you are getting enough of the vital nutrients like vitamin B12, calcium, and vitamin D, you should include fortified foods in your diet. Some examples of these foods are plant milks, morning cereals, and nutritional yeast.

5. *Supplementation:* If you believe that your food consumption may be insufficient, you should evaluate the possibility of taking vitamin B12 and vitamin D supplements. When determining specific requirements, it is best to confer with a healthcare practitioner.

6. *Devote a certain amount of time* each

week to the process of meal preparation and cooking in bulk. In order to simplify the process of preparing meals during the hectic weekdays, it is helpful to prepare essentials such as grains, beans, and roasted vegetables in advance.

7. *Experiment with different recipes* and cooking techniques to make meals interesting and pleasurable for the entire family. This may be accomplished by becoming creative with recipes. In order to cultivate a healthy connection with food, it is important to engage children in the process of meal planning and preparation.

You can make certain that your family obtains the necessary nutrients to survive on a plant-based diet by adhering to these principles and ensuring that they are-implemented.

It is vital to have a fundamental grasp of the nutritional components of a plant-based diet in order to keep one's health and well-being at their highest possible level. You are able to offer your family with well-balanced, nutritious meals that are beneficial to their overall health and vitality if you address dietary shortages, place an emphasis on plant foods that are high in nutrients, and use smart tactics for meal planning.

3

This is the hidden weapon that every successful plant-based chef has at their disposal: a well-stocked pantry. In this chapter, we will discuss how to effectively fill your pantry with vital components in order to improve the flavor of your meals as well as the health advantages they provide. If you want to make sure that your path toward a plant-based diet is not only tasty but also sustainable, we will also discuss buying tactics that are kind to your wallet and ways to reduce the amount of food that is wasted.

Tips for Stocking a Pantry That Is Based on Plants

1. *"Variety is the Key":* In order to optimize both your nutritional intake and your culinary inventiveness, you should strive to consume a wide variety of entire foods, such as grains, legumes,

nuts, seeds, fruits, and vegetables.
2. When it comes to maintaining maximum nutrition and taste in your recipes, it is important to *prioritize whole foods* and choose components that have undergone minimum processing.

3. *Read the labels:* When purchasing packaged goods, it is important to be aware of any undetected additives and preservatives. Pick items that have components that are easy to recognize and uncomplicated.

Essential Components and the Diverse Applications They Bring
1. *Quinoa, brown rice, and oats* are an example of grains that may be used as diverse foundation for salads, bowls, and breakfast items.

2. *Legumes,* which include chickpeas, black beans, and lentils, are a source of protein that may be added to plant-

based burgers, stews, and soups by adding them.

3. *Nuts and seeds:* Almonds, chia seeds, and flaxseeds are examples of nuts and seeds that enrich smoothies, salads, and baked products with beneficial fats and different textures.

4. *Garlic, cumin, and turmeric* are examples of herbs and spices that may be used to enhance the taste of sauces, stir-fries, and curries.

The following are some strategies for shopping on a budget and reducing the amount of food that is wasted:

1. *Make a plan ahead of time:* Make a weekly meal plan and a shopping list to prevent yourself from making impulsive purchases and to guarantee that you only buy what you need.

2. *Buy in Bulk:* If you want to save money and limit the amount of trash that is produced by packing, you should

buy essentials like grains, beans, and spices in bulk.

3. *Acknowledge and Embrace Imperfection:* Do not be afraid to purchase things that are reduced or produce that has a small imperfection. Both in terms of their nutritional value and their ability to be converted into delectable dishes.

If you follow these guidelines and fill your pantry with healthful plant-based products, you will be well-equipped to prepare nutritional meals that will satisfy your taste senses and support your efforts to achieve your health objectives. Joy in the kitchen!

4

Put yourself in the position of a small kid who joyfully assists their parent in the preparation of supper. There is a gleam of enthusiasm in their eyes as they meticulously slice the bright veggies and joyously sprinkle the spices into the saucepan. This youngster is not only assisting; rather, they are really engrossed in the process, and they are ecstatic at the possibility of producing something that is both tasty and wholesome. The significance of fostering a passion for healthy nutrition in children at an early age is shown by this scenario, which is both uplifting and inspiring.

Ideas for meals that are both creative and nutritious

1. *"Rainbow Veggie Wraps"*: Instruct children to make their own wraps by using tortillas made from nutritious

grains and filling them with a variety of colorful vegetables such as bell peppers, cucumbers, carrots, and spinach. Include hummus or avocado for an additional layer of flavor and richness.

2. *To make quesadillas with sweet potatoes and black beans,* mash roasted sweet potatoes with black beans and put the mixture between two tortillas made with healthy grains. After being grilled until they are crispy, serve them with salsa and guacamole for dipping.

3. *Small Veggie Pizzas:* Give children the opportunity to construct their very own small pizzas by creating the foundation out of pita bread or English muffins made with whole wheat. There should be a selection of toppings available, including tomato sauce, sliced bell peppers, mushrooms, olives, and cheese that does not contain dairy.

4. *To make a thick smoothie foundation,* freeze mixed berries, banana, and plant-based milk are blended together in a blender. This recipe is for fruit smoothie bowls. It should be poured into bowls, and then granola, sliced fruit, shredded coconut, and a drizzle of nut butter should be sprinkled on top.

5. In order to make *crunchy vegetable nuggets,* first coat cauliflower or broccoli florets in a combination of breadcrumbs and nutritional yeast, and then bake them until they are fully coated. Served with a serving of ketchup or barbecue sauce that you have created yourself.

Methods for Including Children in the Process of Preparing Breakfast and Lunch
1. Involve children in the process of meal planning by *allowing them to choose fruits, veggies,* and other items at the grocery store or farmer's market. This will allow them to take active

participation in the process. 2. *Give children age-appropriate jobs to do.* For example, you may give kids easy chores like as cleaning fruit, stirring ingredients, or placing toppings on pizzas. This will help them feel like they are contributing to the process.

3. In order to make the process of preparing meals more enjoyable, *you may turn it into a game or an activity that requires creativity* by giving things humorous names or promoting imaginative play in the kitchen.

Fostering a Positive Relationship with Food

1. *Serve as a model for others to follow* by demonstrating a willingness to experiment with different cuisines and highlighting the enjoyment of consuming a wide range of healthy foods.

2. *Establish Encouragement Routines*

for Your Mealtimes: Establishing a relaxing and pleasurable atmosphere at mealtimes may be accomplished by sitting down as a family, exchanging tales, and expressing thanks for the food that is set before you.

You will be able to encourage your children to establish good eating habits and a positive connection with food that will serve them well throughout their lives if you include these tactics and meal ideas into the routine that your family follows.

5

The benefits of meal prepping, which include saving time, are a surprising fact.

Did you know that preparing meals ahead of time can save hard-working families an average of eight to ten hours per week? This seemingly insignificant routine has the potential to make a significant difference in terms of lowering stress levels and increasing productivity in day-to-day life. When families spend just a few hours on the weekend preparing meals, they are able to take advantage of the convenience of having meals that are already prepared and ready to eat throughout the week. This allows them to devote more time to other activities.

1. *Schedule "Sunday Prep Sessions":* Set aside a particular time each week, such as the afternoon of Sunday, to take care of the preparation of meals. Make use of this time to prepare meals in containers, chop vegetables, and cook grains and proteins at the same time. This will allow you to easily grab and go meals during the hectic weekdays.

2. Create *"Sheet Pan Dinners"* to simplify the process of meal preparation by cooking all of the meals on a single sheet pan. It is recommended that you select a protein, such as chicken or tofu, and then combine it with the vegetables and seasoning of your choice. By roasting everything together, you can make a meal that is both delicious and nutritious, and it only requires a small amount of cleanup.

3. Utilize the power of the Instant Pot to prepare meals in a quick and effective manner by *utilizing the Instant Pot's versatility*. Dishes such as chili, curry, or risotto can be prepared in a fraction of the time that they would take to prepare directly on the stovetop. Prepare large quantities of food in bulk and then freeze individual portions for use in subsequent meals.

4. *Mason Jar Salads:* To make salads that are portable, you can make them in mason jars by layering ingredients such as dressing, grains, protein, vegetables, and leafy greens. These salads are ready-made and can be stored in the refrigerator for several days without losing their freshness. They are ideal for packing in lunchboxes or for enjoying as a speedy and nutritious dinner option.

The Importance of Cooking in Batches for the Success of Mealtimes on a Regular Basis

A game-changer for busy families who are striving for consistent success during mealtimes is the ability to cook in batches. Families are able to streamline the cooking process and ensure that healthy options are always available by preparing large batches of staple ingredients such as grains, beans, and roasted vegetables in advance. This allows for constant availability of nutritious options. By allowing for flexibility in meal planning and encouraging creativity in the use of leftovers to create new and exciting dishes, batch cooking also allows for greater flexibility.

Meal prepping and cooking in bulk are indispensable tools for busy families who are striving to maintain a healthy and balanced lifestyle despite the hectic schedules they frequently find themselves in. You will be able to save time, reduce stress, and enjoy delicious homemade meals together as a family if you incorporate these strategies and recipes into your daily routine.

6

Amazing Information Regarding the Positive Effects That Herbs and Spices Have on One's Health

1. *Anti-Inflammatory characteristics:* Numerous herbs and spices, including turmeric, ginger, and cinnamon, have powerful anti-inflammatory characteristics that may assist in reducing inflammation inside the body. This can possibly lessen the chance of developing chronic illnesses such as arthritis and heart disease.

2. *The abundance of antioxidants:* Herbs and spices are loaded with antioxidants, which help neutralize potentially damaging free radicals and protect cells from damage. Some examples of spices that are especially high in antioxidants are cloves, oregano, and cinnamon. These spices all

contribute to general health and well-being.

3. *Digestive Support:* Certain herbs and spices, such as ginger and peppermint, may help with digestion by decreasing bloating, gas, and indigestion respectively. In addition to this, they have the ability to accelerate the synthesis of digestive enzymes, which results in improved nutritional absorption.

A Wide Range of Herbs and Spices That Were Typically Employed in Plant-Based Cooking

1. *Turmeric:* This spice, which is well-known for its bright yellow color and earthy taste, includes curcumin, a molecule that has potent anti-inflammatory and antioxidant qualities. This gives rice dishes, soups, and curries a more complex flavor.

2. *Cinnamon:* This sweet and fragrant

spice is not only tasty, but it also helps manage blood sugar levels and increase insulin sensitivity. Cinnamon is a spice that has sweet and aromatic properties. It is a healthful and tasty addition that may be sprinkled over toppings such as fruit, yogurt, or oatmeal.

3. *Basil*, which has a flavor that is both fresh and somewhat spicy, is an essential ingredient in the cuisine of the Mediterranean region. It adds a healthy dose of vitamin K and a burst of flavor to salads, pasta, and tomatoes, and it goes nicely with all of these dishes.

Recipes and suggestions for incorporating herbs and spices into meals that are consumed on a daily basis
1. To make a delectable and healthy alternative to regular rice, *try making turmeric cauliflower rice* by sautéing grated cauliflower with turmeric, cumin, and garlic. These may be used as a basis for Buddha bowls or as a side dish.

2. *Cooking oats with almond milk, cinnamon, and chopped apples* results in a breakfast that is both comforting and satiating. Consider making cinnamon apple oatmeal. As an additional indulgence, garnish with a drizzle of maple syrup and a topping of nuts.

3. *To produce a pesto sauce that is both vivid and savory,* you may prepare basil pesto pasta by blending together fresh basil, garlic, pine nuts, olive oil, and nutritional yeast via a blender. Cooked spaghetti and cherry tomatoes may be tossed together to create a supper that is both fast and tasty.

You may improve the taste of your plant-based meals by adding herbs and spices to them, which not only increases their nutritional content but also improves their flavor. Experiment with a variety of different combinations to find the taste profiles that you like the most and to realize the myriad health advantages that these combinations bring.

7

Plant-Based Protein Sources for Optimal Health

Eradicating Common Misconceptions Regarding Protein Derived from Plants

1. *Erroneous belief:* proteins derived from plants are of lower quality than proteins derived from animals. The reality is that when taken in sufficient quantities and from a variety of sources, proteins derived from plants have the potential to provide all of the essential amino acids that are required for human health.

2. It is a common misconception that a *plant-based diet makes it harder to satisfy one's need for protein.* The truth is that, Protein may be found in abundance in a wide variety of plant-based foods, and it is fully possible to fulfill one's protein needs only via the consumption of plant-based foods if one

makes the necessary preparations.

Various Plant-Based Protein Sources and the Nutritional Benefits associated with Each-of-Them

1. *Beans, lentils, and chickpeas* are all great sources of protein, fiber, vitamins, and minerals. Additionally, legumes are a good source of fiber. The versatility of these ingredients allows them to be used in a wide variety of recipes, including soups, stews, salads, and burgers.

2. The following are examples of nuts and seeds: *almonds, chia seeds, and hemp seeds* are all rich in protein, healthy fats, and minerals such as magnesium and zinc. Mixing them into smoothies, cereal, and homemade energy bars is a fantastic way to incorporate them.

3. *Quinoa, brown rice, and oats* are examples of whole grains. These grains are rich in protein, fiber, and complex

carbs, and they are also a source of complex carbohydrates. They are the foundation of a wide variety of plant-based dishes, including salads, stir-fries, and grain bowls, among others.

Instructions on How to Satisfy Your Needs for-Protein

1. *Whole Foods:* Place an emphasis on integrating a range of plant-based protein sources into each meal. For example, using beans in conjunction with rice or using nuts and seeds in salads are both examples of this. Strive to consume a diet that is well-balanced and abundant in fruits, vegetables, legumes, and whole grains.

2. *Plant-Based Protein Supplements:* Although they are not always required, protein supplements may be helpful for persons who have elevated protein demands. Some examples of these individuals are athletes and people who adhere to a vegan diet religiously. Be on

the lookout for plant-based protein powders of superior quality that are produced from sources such as pea, hemp, or brown rice beans.

Plant-based sources of protein provide a multitude of health advantages and are simple to add into a diet that meets the requirements of a balanced diet. Individuals may live on a plant-based diet while still fulfilling their protein requirements if they make a conscious effort to vary their food choices and pay attention to their nutritional requirements.

8

The Role of Whole Grains in Plant-Based Nutrition

*"Whole grains are a nutritional powerhouse, offering a wealth of health benefits that support overall well-being". If you want to enhance your digestion, increase your energy levels, and lower your chance of developing chronic illnesses, include whole grains in your diet is quite beneficial.**

An Understanding of the Significance of Whole-Grains

Due to the abundant nutritional profile that they provide, whole grains are an essential component of a well-balanced plant-based diet. As a result of their high fiber content, vitamin and mineral content, and antioxidant content, they provide a multitude of health advantages. Whole grains include fiber, which is beneficial to digestive health, helps control blood sugar levels, and contributes to the maintenance of a healthy weight. Furthermore, there is a correlation between the consumption of whole grains and a decreased risk of cardiovascular disease, stroke, type 2 diabetes, and some malignancies.

Incorporating Whole Grains into Your Diet When You Follow a Plant-Based Diet
1. *The Quinoa Salad with Roasted Vegetables* is the first meal. Prepare the quinoa in accordance with the directions provided on the box, and then combine it with roasted vegetables such as cherry tomatoes, bell peppers, and zucchini. Lemon vinaigrette is a delightful condiment that may be drizzled over the food.

2. *Cook brown rice and stir-fry* it with tofu, broccoli, carrots, and snap peas in a tasty sauce made from soy sauce, garlic, and ginger. This dish is referred to as brown rice stir-fry.

3. *Onions, garlic, and spices such as cumin, coriander,* and cinnamon should be sautéed in the pan before adding the chickpeas and bulgur to the dish. Include chickpeas, bulgur that has been cooked, and vegetable broth. Using fresh herbs as a garnish, simmer the mixture until all of the liquid has been absorbed.

Techniques for Cooking with Whole Grains

1. Before you cook the grains, you should rinse them to eliminate any dirt and to enhance their texture.

2. For the majority of types, adhere to a water-to-grain ratio of two to one.

3. Conduct experiments using a variety of culinary techniques, including boiling, steaming, and baking, among others.

4. Maintaining the freshness of whole grains requires that they be stored in sealed containers in a cold, dry location.

Whole grains are an essential component of plant-based nutrition since they provide a wide range of advantages to one's health and may be used in a variety of ways in the kitchen. You may improve the taste of your meals as well as the nutritional worth of your meals by include a range of whole grains in your diet.

9

Did you know that vegetables and other plant-based products provide a degree of variety in the culinary arts that is unmatched by any other? In the realm of plant-based cuisine, there is a plethora of different and interesting tastes just waiting to be discovered. These flavors range from vivid vegetables to robust legumes and fragrant herbs and spices.

Investigating Different Methods for Improvement of Flavor

1. *Using Umami:* Umami, sometimes referred to as the fifth taste, has the ability to enhance the flavor of foods that are based on plant-based ingredients. If you want to give your dishes more depth and complexity, try including umami-rich items like mushrooms, tomatoes, miso paste, and soy sauce into your eating routine.

2. *Acidic components*, such as citrus juices, vinegar, and fermented foods, have the ability to enhance the tastes of plant-based cuisine. This is referred to as "balancing acidity." Make use of them in moderation to achieve a balance between sweetness and richness, as well as to provide a revitalizing zing to your dishes.

3. *Layering Spices and Herbs:* If you want to develop layers of taste in your recipes, try experimenting with a wide selection of spices and herbs. Enhancing the scent and strength of spices may be accomplished by toasting them before using them. When it comes to developing powerful flavor profiles, you shouldn't be afraid to experiment with bold combos such as cumin and coriander or rosemary and thyme.

Useful Advice for Creating Flavorful Foods Using Plant-Based Ingredients
1. *Try out a variety of cooking*

techniques by experimenting with them: In order to bring out the inherent tastes of plant-based products and to produce a more complex flavor profile, you should experiment with cooking methods such as roasting, grilling, sautéing, and braising.

2. *Balance tastes and Textures:* Aim for a harmonic balance of tastes (sweet, sour, salty, bitter, and umami) and textures (crispy, creamy, chewy, and crunchy) in your meals to keep them interesting and fulfilling.

3. *Experiment with unorthodox spices* like as nutritional yeast, smoky paprika, or tahini to add new and interesting taste aspects to your foods. Don't be afraid to look outside the box and experiment with unconventional seasonings.

Being an expert in the art of gourmet plant-based cooking requires embracing the plethora of resources that are accessible and making use of a variety of methods and spices in order to produce meals that are both delicious and gratifying, while also celebrating the diversity of plant-based cuisine for its diversity.

10

Navigating Social Situations and Dining Out

Living a plant-based lifestyle may provide its own set of obstacles, particularly in social contexts where dietary habits may be different from culture to culture. In this article, we will discuss some of the most frequent difficulties that families who adhere to a plant-based diet experience when they are in social settings, as well as some successful solutions for eating out while still practicing a plant-based lifestyle.

Common Obstacles to Overcome in Social Establishments

1. *Limited Menu alternatives:* Many social events may not include plant-based menu alternatives, which may leave persons who strictly adhere to a plant-based diet feeling excluded or forcing them to make food choices that are not appropriate.

2. *Social Pressure:* Family get-togethers or celebrations with friends sometimes contain traditional cuisines that may not be compatible with a plant-based diet. This might result in social pressure to indulge in foods that are not derived from plants.

Methods to Consider When Eating Out
1. *Before going out to eat,* do some research on restaurants that provide plant-based alternatives or give them a call in advance to ask about the availability of menu items that are suitable for plant-based diets.

2. *"Customize Your Order":* Do not be afraid to request that menu items be modified in order to make them suitable for plant-based diets. The vast majority of eateries are ready to accommodate customers' dietary needs.

3. *Look for Restaurants That Serve Plant-Based Foods:* If you want to have a satisfactory eating experience, you should look for restaurants that either specialize in plant-based cuisine or offer a broad variety of plant-based alternatives.

What You Should Know About Communicating Your Dietary Preferences
1. *Make sure that your dietary choices are communicated* to the hosts or the personnel at the restaurant in a way that is both courteous and forceful. This will guarantee that your requirements are satisfied.

2. *Offer to Bring a meal:* When you go to social events, make it a point to offer to bring a meal that is made from plant-based ingredients to share. This will ensure that there is something that you can enjoy and will also introduce people to great plant-based alternatives.

3. *Educate Others:* Make the most of the chance to educate your friends and family about the advantages of a plant-based diet and the ways in which they may support your dietary choices.

The ability to successfully navigate social settings and eat out while sticking to a plant-based diet takes careful preparation, assertiveness, and the ability to communicate effectively. Individuals who follow a plant-based diet may successfully handle social events while adhering to their dietary choices if they put these ideas and recommendations into practice.

11

The Mindfulness Exercise That Is Engaging

First, let's take a minute to participate in a simple mindfulness exercise before we get into the practice of mindful eating. Take a few deep breaths, close your eyes, and focus your attention on the feelings that are occurring inside your body. Take note of the rate at which you breathe, the sensation of your feet on the ground, and the noises that are occurring in your environment. Now, return your attention to the here and now in a gentle manner, letting go of any ideas or distractions that may be distracting you. After taking another deep breath, you should open your eyes when you feel ready to do so.

Advantages of Practicing Mindful Eating

1. *Enhanced Awareness:* The practice of

mindful eating teaches us to pay special attention to the sensory experience of eating, which includes the taste, the texture, and the smell of the food themselves. We are able to more perfectly taste and appreciate our meals when we are totally present.

2. *The practice of eating consciously* enables us to become more in touch with our body's signals of hunger and fullness, which in turn leads to improved digestion and a decreased likelihood of overeating or experiencing pain in the digestive tract.

3. Mindful eating helps us develop a *non-judgmental awareness* of our feelings and eating patterns, which is an important step in the process of emotional regulation. It is possible to cultivate healthy connections with food and better control emotional eating if we allow ourselves to observe our thoughts and emotions without attaching

ourselves   to   them.
The following are some methods for cultivating mindfulness when eating with your-family

1. One way to promote sensory awareness is to encourage members of the family to *engage their senses while they are eating* by describing the colors, textures, and tastes of the food they are eating. Both the appreciation for the food and the habits of mindful eating may be strengthened as a result of this.

2. Instruct everyone to eat slowly and to relish each mouthful by following the *"Slow Down"* instruction. In order to allow for sufficient time for pleasure and digestion, it is important to encourage discussion and connection during meals.

3. Before each meal, encourage every member of the family to express thanks for the food that was prepared and the work that was put into making it. This is an example of the *thankfulness practice.*

A feeling of gratitude and mindfulness is developed as a result of this practice at mealtimes.

4. When it comes to mindful portion control, it is important to *teach both children and adults* to pay attention to their bodies and stop eating when they are content. This is in contrast to the common practice of completing everything on their plate out of habit or duty.

We can cultivate a culture of present, gratitude, and well-being around food by implementing these mindful eating practices into family meals. This will nurture not just our bodies but also our relationships with one another.

12

Examples of Athletes Overcoming Obstacles to Achieve Success on Plant-Based Diets

1. *Scott Jurek,* an ultra-marathoner, attributes his extraordinary stamina and repeated victories in ultra-running events to the fact that he follows a plant-based diet.

2. *Serena Williams:* Tennis great Serena Williams consumes a plant-based diet in order to fuel her strenuous training sessions and to ensure that she continues to perform at her highest level on the court.

3. *Lewis Hamilton:* Formula One winner Lewis Hamilton credits his success on the racetrack to his plant-based diet, which he feels improves both

his physical and emotional well-being. Hamilton is a plant-based vegan.

The Scientific Implications of Plant-Based Dietary Supplements for Physical Performance and Recuperation
1. *Nutrient Density:* Plant-based diets are abundant in vital nutrients, such as complex carbohydrates, antioxidants, vitamins, and minerals, which are responsible for providing prolonged energy and supporting the repair of muscles.

2. *Anti-Inflammatory Properties:* Numerous plant foods, including fruits, vegetables, nuts, and seeds, include anti-inflammatory substances that have the ability to decrease inflammation that is caused by exercise and promote a more rapid recovery.

3. Plant-based diets are connected with *higher blood flow and cardiovascular health,* which may boost oxygen supply

to muscles during exercise, hence enhancing performance and lowering tiredness. This is one of the benefits of plant-based diets.

Guidance on how to maximize the nutritional intake of active members of the family

1. *Consume a Wide Range of Consumable Plant-Based Foods:* To ensure that your family receives all of the important nutrients for maximum performance and development, you should encourage them to eat a wide variety of fruits, vegetables, whole grains, legumes, nuts, and seeds.

2. It is vital to incorporate *protein-rich foods* such as tofu, tempeh, lentils, beans, and quinoa in order to promote muscle repair and development. Although plant-based diets may supply an acceptable quantity of protein, it is essential to prioritize the sources of protein.

3. The importance of *maintaining enough hydration* cannot be overstated when it comes to both physical performance and recuperation. Be sure to encourage the members in your family to consume a sufficient amount of water throughout the day, particularly before, during, and after physical activity.

4. *Plan Balanced Meals:* In order to promote energy levels, muscular function, and general well-being, it is important to plan balanced meals that contain a variety of carbs, protein, healthy fats, and micronutrients.

It is possible for members of an active family, including children and teenagers, to reach their performance objectives and flourish physically if they adhere to these rules and adopt a plant-based diet that is abundant in foods that are rich in nutrients.

13

Managing Weight and Promoting Healthy Growth

There is a rising worry all over the globe over the issue of childhood obesity, which has long-term ramifications for health and well-being. Recent figures indicate that there were around 38 million children under the age of five who were either overweight or obese in the year 2020, and the prevalence of these conditions is gradually being on the rise. In light of the fact that obesity in children is linked to a variety of health problems, including diabetes, cardiovascular disease, stroke, and cancer, this trend is quite concerning.

Strategies for Managing Weight and Promoting Healthy Growth through Plant-Based-Nutrition.

1. Put all of your attention on whole, *plant-based foods:* It is important to encourage youngsters to eat a wide

variety of foods, including fruits, vegetables, legumes, nuts, seeds, and whole grains. The high levels of fiber, vitamins, minerals, and antioxidants that are included in these foods contribute to feelings of fullness and general health.

2. *Reduce Your Intake of Processed meals and Sugary Drinks:* Reduce the amount of processed meals, sugary snacks, and drinks that are especially rich in added sugars that you consume. The use of these things contributes to an excessive amount of calories, which might result in weight gain.

3. *Encourage regular physical exercise:* In order to promote weight control and general health, it is important to encourage regular physical activity. Children should be encouraged to participate in activities that they love, such as dancing, playing outside, or participating in sports.

4. *Instruct children to make mindful eating* a habit by teaching them to pay attention to their hunger and fullness signals and to eat in a thoughtful manner. Inspire them to eat slowly, to relish the food they are eating, and to pay attention to the signals that their body sends them about hunger and fullness.

5. *Involve Children in Meal Preparation:* Involve children in the process of planning and preparing meals in order to encourage their enthusiasm in eating healthily. Give kids the opportunity to choose fruits and vegetables at the grocery store and to participate in the preparation of simple meals.

Practical Approaches to Assist in Meeting the Nutritional Requirements of Children
1. *Infants (ages 0 to 12 months):* - It is advised that infants be breastfed for the

first six months of their lives, after which they should be introduced to solid meals that are high in nutrients.
- In order to provide a range of tastes and textures, you should provide a selection of purees and mashed meals that have just one component.

2. *In the early years of childhood (ages 1 to-5),* A diet that is well-balanced should be provided, and it should consist of a wide range of fruits, vegetables, whole grains, lean meats, and healthy fats.
- Provide them with regular, little meals and snacks in order to satisfy their energy requirements and to encourage their growth and development.

3. *Middle childhood, which spans from 6 to-11-years:* Continue to promote a diet that is well-balanced and has an emphasis on foods that are high in nutrients.
- Instruction should be given to

youngsters on the significance of selecting nutritious foods and the advantages of engaging in regular physical exercise.

4. Supporting adolescents in making well-informed decisions about the foods they consume and establishing healthy eating habits is an important aspect of *adolescence-(12-18-years)*.

They should be encouraged to engage in sports and other activities that they love, as well as to be physically active throughout their time.

Through the implementation of these measures and the provision of assistance at each stage of development, parents are able to assist their children in managing their weight, fostering healthy growth, and establishing habits that will last a lifetime, such as eating nutritious foods and engaging in regular physical exercise.

14

Inspiring Anecdotes Regarding the Adoption of a Plant-Based Lifestyle

1. *"The Smith Family's Journey":* The Smiths, a family of four, decided to go on a plant-based journey after they had been struggling with issues related to their weight and their health. They were able to achieve weight loss, increased energy levels, and an overall improvement in their well-being by adopting a diet that consisted of plant-based foods and whole foods. Their experience is illustrative of the positive effects that can be achieved through the consumption of plant-based foods.

2. *"The Johnsons' Health Transformation":* The Johnson family made the decision to adopt a plant-based lifestyle because they wanted to

reduce their risk of developing chronic diseases and live a life that was more environmentally friendly. They were successful in lowering their cholesterol levels, reducing inflammation, and improving their immune system by consuming a diet that was primarily composed of plant-based foods. Others were motivated to adopt their newfound vitality and resiliency as a result of their example.

The Overcoming of Obstacles and the Maintenance of a Plant-Based Lifestyle
1. *Planning and preparing meals:* in the first place Devote some of your time to the planning and preparation of meals in order to guarantee a wide range of wholesome plant-based meals. During the hectic weekdays, the process can be simplified and time saved by using recipes that are freezer-friendly and can be prepared in bulk.

2. *"Navigating Social Situations":* In

order to be ready for social gatherings, you should bring plant-based dishes to share with others or communicate your dietary preferences to the hosts in advance. Rather than allowing yourself to feel constrained by the food choices you make, focus on the joy of connecting with loved ones.

3. *Addressing Concerns Regarding Nutriten Content:* Through the consumption of fortified foods, supplements, and a varied diet consisting of plant-based foods, you can ensure that you are getting an adequate amount of essential nutrients such as vitamin B12, iron, calcium, and omega-3 fatty acids. Making an appointment with a registered dietitian can provide you with individualized advice.

4. *To maintain your motivation,* look for ideas in plant-based cookbooks, documentaries, online communities, and success stories. This will help you

stay motivated. Celebrate even the smallest of victories and concentrate on the positive changes that have occurred in your health and well-being.

Support and Resources for Those Who Are Taking a Plant-Based Diet

1. *Cookbooks and Recipe Websites:* If you are looking for creative and delectable meal ideas, you should start by looking through plant-based cookbooks and recipe websites. Forks Over Knives, Oh She Glows, and Minimalist Baker are just a few examples of websites that provide a plethora of plant-based recipes that are suitable for any occasion.

2. *Online Communities and Support Groups:* Join online communities and support groups dedicated to plant-based living. Facebook groups and the r/PlantBasedDiet subreddit on Reddit are two examples of platforms that offer a space for individuals to discuss their

experiences, pose questions, and seek support from others who share similar perspectives.

3. *Educational Resources:* Educate yourself about the science behind plant-based nutrition by reading books, watching documentaries, and visiting websites that have a good reputation. Several resources, including "Forks Over Knives," "The Game Changers," and NutritionFacts.org, provide information that is supported by evidence regarding the positive effects that plant-based diets have on one's health.

Through the implementation of these strategies and the utilization of the resources and support that are readily available, individuals and families are able to effortlessly incorporate plant-based nutrition into their day-to-day lives, which ultimately results in enhanced health outcomes and a lifestyle that is more sustainable.

15

A Retrospective on the Procedures Taken to Achieve Better Health

As you embark on the road of plant-based nutrition, you are not just making a change to your diet; you are also embarking on a transforming journey toward improved health and energy. During the process of transitioning to a plant-based diet, families often become aware of significant changes in their overall health. In addition to better digestion and weight control, the advantages are many and significant. These benefits include enhanced levels of energy. When we take the time to reflect on our journey, we are able to see the wonderful changes that have occurred and reaffirm our determination to put the health of our family first.

1. *The Johnson Family:* The Johnsons saw tremendous gains in their general health after making the decision to move to a plant-based diet. Mrs. Johnson had a considerable reduction in the frequency and severity of her severe migraines, while Mr. Johnson's cholesterol readings returned to normal limits. During the time that they spent together in the kitchen and eating meals, their children encountered less incidences of sickness and allergies, and the closeness that they enjoyed with one another further deepened.

2. *The Smith Family:* The Smiths' path to plant-based eating started with skepticism, but it rapidly grew into a lifestyle that they couldn't think how they would live without. Together, they were able to lose extra weight, reverse the progression of prediabetes, and discover the delight that comes from

experimenting with new tastes and ingredients. The transformational impact of plant-based nourishment for the whole family is shown by their tale, which stands as a witness to this power.

Providing Some Closing Words of Comfort and-Encouragement

During this time of celebration for our plant-based journey's accomplishments and landmarks, let us not forget that maintaining good health is a quest that lasts a lifetime. Each and every baby step that we take toward improved nutrition and overall health is a contribution to the long-term vitality of our family. Maintain your dedication to providing your loved ones with healthful plant-based meals, with the knowledge that you are establishing the groundwork for a future that is both healthier and happier for the two of you. Accept the journey, rejoice in your accomplishments, and keep putting the well-being and vitality of your family at the forefront of your priorities above all-else.

Let us make the most of the time we spend together at the dinner table, appreciating the delectable plant-based meals that not only feed our bodies but also our spirits. Every member of our family should experience happiness, appreciation, and an abundance of well-being as they travel the path toward health and vitality. May this trip be prosperous.

Conclusion

"Harvesting Health: Plant-Based Nutrition Secrets for Happy Families" talks about how plant-based nutrition can change families' health and energy for the better. Important things to remember from the book are:

1. *Health Benefits:* Plant-based meals have many health benefits, such as making you healthier, giving you more energy, improving digestion, helping you lose weight, and lowering your risk of getting chronic diseases.

2. *Sustainability:* Living a plant-based lifestyle helps the earth by lowering your carbon footprint and keeping natural resources from being used up.

3. *Family Bonding:* Making and eating plant-based food together can improve family ties and make everyone feel more connected.

4. *Longevity:* A plant-based diet can help you live longer and be healthier overall, so your family can do well and enjoy life to the best.

Plant-based eating is clearly not only good for your health but also important for keeping your family happy and healthy. Because of this, it is very important for people to start their road to health with joy and confidence. Families can take care of their health, protect the environment, and leave a legacy of wellness for future generations by putting plant-based foods first. Let's trust the power of plants and start this journey together, knowing that each step will bring us closer to a better, happy future.